AFRICAN AMERICAN OLD HOME REMEDIES

The Legacy And Home Remedies Of My

Family's Ancient Healers

Written & Compiled By
Rev. Dr. Geraldine L. Carter

"A healer's power stems not from any special ability, but from maintaining the courage and awareness to embody and express the universal healing power that every human being naturally possesses."

-Eric Micha'el Leventhal

any usage or abuse of any policies, processes, or directions contained within is the solitary and utter responsibility of the recipient reader. Under no circumstances will any legal responsibility or blame be held against the publisher for any reparation, damages, or monetary loss due to the information herein, either directly or indirectly.

Respective authors own all copyrights not held by the publisher. The information herein is offered for informational purposes solely, and is universal as so. The presentation of the information is without contract or any type of guarantee assurance.

The trademarks that are used are without any consent, and the publication of the trademark is without permission or backing by the trademark owner. All trademarks and brands within this book are for clarifying purposes only and are then owned by the owners themselves, not affiliated with this document.

Table of Contents

PREFACE

This book is written for those who are interested in rediscovering and learning about some of the "Old Home Remedies" used by our grandparents and others who have gone before us.

In the days of old, many had no other options when illness occurred, but to use herbs and natural remedies for themselves and those who came to them for the "cure". Herbs and other remedies were used also, to prevent illness and disease.

The descriptive information is written mostly from my memory of my Grandmother, but even more so, from the memory of my Great-Grandmother, both of whom I have come to realize played a very important role in who I am, and who I am becoming today.

What I was unable to recall, I begged, pleaded, and coaxed out of my mother, Girthel Johnson-Bryant's memory of her Mother and Grandmother. There are a few other people who knew and were close to my Grandmother and they have contributed also.

One of those special people who contributed to this information is Walter Rowles, who found a notebook that belonged to my grandmother with many of these herbal cures inside. So Thank you to those souls who are now in heaven.

It is important for me to tell the story of the practices of my Grandmother and Great-Grandmother to give credit to where these home remedies came from. They were African American Healers and I want to honor them by introducing them to you before I go into the remedies.

It is important for you to know about and use these remedies if you desire, but please do not allow them to serve as a replacement for professional medical care. They are not meant to be used without a full knowledge of the side effects as well.

Listen to your body and pay close attention to how your body reacts to herbs, and then adjust your use of them accordingly. So please, always use discretion and be aware that the application of home remedies in this book is **AT YOUR OWN RISK**.

Not everything will work the same for everyone, and your mind will always be the greatest healer you will ever be in contact with. That's because the mind and the body are connected in more ways than we and even medical professionals truly understand.

For me, this is a spiritual journey of stepping back in time and reliving the herbal healing practices of my Grandmothers. And it is my pleasure to share this journey with you, along with sharing some "secret" healing techniques that have been passed down to me.

I wish you well!

Rev. Dr. Geraldine Johnson-Carter

INTRODUCTION

I am pleased to be able to provide an introduction to my grandmother's and grandmother's old home remedies which were similar to many that I learned from the healers in Belize, Central America and in Caribbean islands of St. Vincent.

Later in my adult life I had the privilege to travel to Central and South America to the Country of Belize, and the Caribbean islands of St. Vincent in the West Indies. There I lived and studied with Black Carib and Garifuna healers.

Many of the remedies I learned that you will read about come from farmers, producers, collectors, herbalists, healers and village women who all have some ideas about plants and foods that can be used as medicine.

The book will be a wonderful reference and resource for those interested in natural healing techniques. I am happy to share what I have learned both in Missouri and from afar with those who are interested in African influenced Home Remedies.

The information from my grandmothers is written mostly from my memory of my Grandmother, but even more so from the memory of my Great Grandmother. Both of whom I have come to realize played a very important role in who I am today.

It was while living in Boonville Missouri taking care of my mother Girthel Johnson-Bryant during the last five years of her life, that I had a chance to spend time talking to her about the memory of her mother, grandmother and a man named Sam Nightingale.

I learned about Sam's spirit and that he was a respected healer in Boonville during the days of slavery. I could feel Sam's spirit while owning and living in a house listed on the national registry of historic places in Boonville.

I was living in Boonville while taking care of my aged mother in what is known as the old "Elenora Penick" home on 312 Spring Street. When I looked at this property that had been vacant for a number of years I felt drawn to it.

It seemed as if I was called to purchase it and set this home up as my work space, and a place to care for my mother until she was moved to Riverdale nursing home in Boonville.

What an enjoyable time I had living and working on Spring Street while taking care of the needs of my Mother. I knew her time was coming to an end, and as her daughter I knew it was my responsibility to be there for her as she was for me in her days of health.

During my time there a dear family friend named Walter Rowles blessed me with a picture of my great grandmother we called mama Birdie, and some brittle, yellow paper with handwritten notes he had saved of herbal cures she used as a traditional healer.

While living on Spring Street, we had many local and out of town visitors. Some of our visitors claimed that they could feel the presence of many spirits in my home. My mother would often say that she could hear a child crying at night.

As for me, I always felt at peace and a sense of belonging in the big house on Spring Street. No one could understand why I wanted the house or felt protected in the large house with four floors and two outer buildings.

I loved the house and I always felt that I was more than welcome being there. Interesting enough, the Mayor of Boonville Bud Kempf at that time would bring people through on tours.

It fascinated him that a woman of color (African American) could own a house where her ancestors had once lived in the slave quarters. Because I could feel the energy of my ancestors, I set up my office and work space in the old slave quarters.

I believe it was because the closeness of the spirit of Sam Nightingale the healer, storyteller and Conjure man, related through blood or spirit that was with me while I lived in Boonville.

During my time in Boonville I learned as much as I could about him. I combined the knowledge of my ancestors Sam Nightingale, my great grandmother Mama Birdie, my grandmother Lottie and my experiences with the healers of Belize and St. Vincent to write this book.

I know for the right people they will take the knowledge I have learned from my ancestors and pass it on as I have. My joy has always been to create and write. So I am passing on their knowledge and legacy to those that wish to receive it. Be well and Blessed in your journey!

Sam Nightingale

Unlike my grandmothers I had to do some research on Sam Nightingale. I found that he had come to Boonville and was a slave of a Dr. Ells from Louisiana, and had lived on many plantations in the South.

Around Boonville Sam was called "Guinea Sam." He claimed to have been shot from a cannon in Africa and ended up in Boonville. Sam walked with a long crooked twisted cane and had a big gold earring.

Because of his time spent around other healers he became the strongest of the "conjure men and women around." It was reported that there was a change in Boonville after Sam arrived.

He was said to have understood both the real and spirit worlds. Guinea Sam claimed he had lived with a southern Indian tribe for several years learning their ways of curing and magic.

The same story was told about African American's living with Indian tribes by my Great-grandfather Charles Leo Johnson's wife who was a full blooded Cherokee Native American.

I met others in my travels outside the U.S.A. both in Belize Central America and St. Vincent that had the same spirit that I believe Sam must have brought with him to Boonville Missouri from West Africa, and left behind for me to find in the 21st Century.

My Grandmother Lottie Bell Henderson

Lottie Bell Henderson carried herself with a quiet dignity and grace. She had a hauntingly strange beauty that came from her Black Irish, African and American Indian heritage.

I have several pictures which show how she looked and dressed in both her young and mature years. "Mama Lottie," as she was called, wore ankle length dresses with crisp white aprons covering them.

Lottie Bell Henderson carried herself with a quiet dignity and grace. She had a hauntingly strange beauty that came from her African and American Indian heritage.

Her hair was completely snow white by the time she was age 50, but it was thick, wavy, cut short and pushed off to one side. She loved to raise chickens, and she was a mid wife who used herbs and plants in the delivery of babies and also for postpartum care of the mothers.

She must have been a brave woman because my mother shared with me how she remembered that her mother would often ride off on horseback through the dark woods at night, just to assist a woman with the delivery of her baby and then ride home again through the dark.

Then before the break of day, she would get up and go to work on her job of cleaning, cooking and washing clothes for the white people in the small town of Bunceton, Missouri.

My mother told me the story of how the woods were full of big, black cats called Panthers. And one night on her way to deliver a baby, Mama Lottie's horse was attacked from the rear by a panther and the horse's rear flank was ripped apart.

Fortunately, Mama Lottie was not far from the house and although there was blood everywhere, the horse was able to make it to the house with Mama Lottie holding on for dear life.

At daybreak she rode back through the same woods, on a different horse of course, but she must have been brave to take the second ride through the woods where her horse had just been attacked.

Grandmother Lottie was a single woman, but not by choice. She wasn't married because my Great Grandmother would not allow any of her three daughters to marry. Because she did not want them to suffer mistreatment at the hands of a husband.

Unfortunately, this was something many black women faced during these times. Once they were married, they were viewed as the property of their husbands to do with as they desired.

The man's ownership over his woman mindset was very similar to the mindset of the slave masters). But the lack of matrimony did not keep Mama Lottie away from men enough to stop her from having children, one of whom was my mother Girthel Redman Johnson- Bryant.

In her day and time, mama Lottie's situation of having children without the benefit of marriage was not unusual for African American women, especially those in the rural South.

The children were often taken care of by the mother and the extended family. In our situation, the main extended family member who was most capable of making a living, was my Great Grandmother mama Birdie.

We all lived together in a small 3 room house. The three adults shared equally in the care and nurturing of the young children. They all also shared the responsibility of working to provide for the family.

Out of the many grandchildren she had, I know that I was my Grandmother's favorite grandchild, because I was small, sickly and also very sassy. Since I was such a sickly child, I required a lot of my Grandmother's attention.

And when she wasn't away from home delivering babies, or caring for the other sick people in our community, I would follow her around asking lots and lots of questions.

I can remember that she liked raising chickens, and she would always carry a garden hoe whenever she went into the chicken coop. She said it was to hoe up the weeds in the garden and if necessary, to kill snakes.

Mama Lottie never smiled much, and now I know why. Life was not easy for her with having so many children to feed and care for. There was no doubt in my mind that she loved her family, and never once regretted having any of her children.

Although she was not as deeply religious as my Great-Grandmother, she was a spiritual person who felt that the only gift that she could give to others, was to give them her nurturing, care, and concern.

As a young child, she taught me many things, through observing her behavior. One thing I remember was that she taught me how to save money, for as she would say "a rainy day".

I used to watch it rain some days and wonder why Mama Lottie would not spend her "rainy day" money. Much of the money that Mama Lottie was saving was the money that one of my uncles, who was in the Army would send her.

She just kept on putting the money in her hiding place so no one else could find it. She hid it so good, that when she died no one could find it. I was too young to remember how to get to the place where her "rainy day" money was hidden.

Mama Lottie also taught me one of the most valuable lessons in humility that I have ever learned. And that lesson is to never look down on another human being, no matter how life has beaten them down.

Often, we would have people who were wandering around the country, looking for work. Since we were just coming out of the Great Depression, they would be looking for food to tide them over until they could find a job.

We never had an over abundance of food, so I never understood how we were able to stretch what little we had, to make it enough to share. So at that young age I was always hungry, so I really wasn't into sharing.

But mama Lottie would not only share our food with strangers, but she would pack a small amount for them to take with them on their journey. When I asked Mama Lottie the questions "Why do we have to share our food with people we don't even know?"

She told me that they would become our extended family and friends. She also said "She would hate to think that one of her children, or grandchildren would ever be somewhere cold and hungry in the world, and no one would feed them."

Now that I have traveled extensively and met many people who were strangers, that have shared their food and their homes with me, I truly know what a valuable lesson it was that she taught me.

My Great Grandmother Burdetta (Birdie) Henderson

Although the memory of my Grandmother mama Lottie is limited, and at times somewhat unclear, the memory of my Great Grandmother Birdie Henderson is very clear. I can even remember quite clearly what she looked like.

She was 5 feet 11 inches tall, and heavy set until her later years when she began to shrink from age. Her skin was the color of rich, warm, caramel. In fact, she often smelled like a caramel apple to me.

Even when she wasn't sitting in her rocking chair by the window, the chair still held her scent and her warmth. I know her smell endearingly because I would often smell the chair when she would move.

One day she caught me. When she asked me why I smelled her chair? I told her it was because it smelled sweet, just like her. She wore braids on the top of her head that were snow white and looked like a crown.

Grandmother Birdie also wore long ankle length dresses, with a stark white full length apron tied around her at all times. She was strong and in her early years, she tipped the scale at around 250 pounds.

My Great Grandma was so strong that everyone respected Miss Birdie Henderson. Her husband, my grandfather was considered as the town "tough guy", and he was the reason that she did not want any of her daughters to get married.

My mother told me that Grandma Birdie felt that they might marry someone just like their father. My grandfather was extremely talented, especially with using a black snake buggy whip as a weapon.

I was told that he once tried to use the whip on my Grandmother. But he only tried once and he did not succeed. After he recovered from the beating she gave him with his own whip, he never tried again.

My Great Grandma Birdie took me under her wing and began to nurture me at a young age. Since I was somewhat frail until I started school, I required special attention for my health.

Birdie Henderson was also a mid wife, and considered to be a master herbalist, because she had knowledge of the healing properties many of the plants that were growing "out back" held behind our small country house in Bunceton, Missouri.

Great Grandmother Birdie knew about various curative plants that most people would never notice or recognize. Some of which she learned about from her mother and older women who lived in our small country town.

She could identify indigenous herbs that her ancestors had used during slavery days, when black people had to depend on themselves and one another for medical treatment.

As a small child I can remember drinking teas brewed from leaves, bark, or roots and poultices made from leaves. There was "goose grease" rubbed on my chest, which was then covered with a warm flannel cloth when I had cold.

I can remember large doses of caster oil and orange juice, which was used to clean out my system when I was sick. To keep all of the children from getting sick, there was the traditional spring tonic, which was a brown liquid that did not smell good

This tonic was administered at the end of the long, cold winter months. We had to hold our nose in order to be able to swallow the spring tonic and keep it down. I never did find out what was in the spring tonic, or what it was supposed to do.

I only knew that when my Grandmother gave it out, there was no escape. We all had to line up and take it or be willing to feel the sting of the braided green switches that she always kept in the corner of her kitchen.

As I reflect back, I do know that when these "natural old home remedies" were used, they often brought about amazing results. I wish I could honestly say that I was a devoted student, and that my grandmother passed on what I now believe was a legacy to me.

Unfortunately, I placed no real value on their wonderful knowledge of herbal remedies, or what is now being called "folk medicine". By the time I began to value their knowledge of using curative plants to heal, both of my potential instructors had passed to the other side of life.

It is only because of my experiences in places where herbs are still being used to remedy a wide range of health problems and maintain good health, that has urged my soul to recognize the value of those women and their gift of healing in my life.

While visiting a small village in Belize Central America, I was told by a very old woman who was also as retired village mid wife about my legacy. Somehow she recognized that I had an unused gift and potential ability to become an herbal and spiritual healer.

She also knew that, up until that specific point in time, I had been involved in activities which did not allow me the time or space to indulge in learning about Nature's healing herbs.

She told me that the time had come for me to accept my gift, and begin to practice the "old ways". She stated that I must "awaken" and recognize the call to act, just as my Grandmothers had, to become a spiritual/herbal healer.

From that meeting and that day on my interest piqued. So I began studying, reading, and talking with anyone who could or would teach me about herbs and "old home remedies".

Just like my ancestors, I now take a holistic approach to health care. This means that I not only treat symptoms using herbs, but I try to discover the reason for and the causes of a person's symptoms.

My Grandmothers understood that being healthy was not only about the health of someone's body, but also the health of an individuals mind and spirit. Because the body, mind and spirit are connected. You can't heal the body without healing the mind.

Both women in my life were positive thinkers, and they always focused on the bright side of life. Which at that time I'm sure must have been difficult for them. Because there were very few material possessions and limited resources.

Prayer, physical exercise, sunshine, water, and rest, played an important role in not only sustaining life for my Grandmothers and their families, but these things were a significant part of the natural treatment methods used for their patients.

My Great Grandma believed in miracles, and when she prayed it was with the conviction that God would answer her prayer and give her the desires of her heart. She was consistent and passionate in her love of God, and she was just as sure of God's love for her.

She and God were a healing team, and the herbs that she used were made more effective because she used them in the name of the Lord. When she prayed, she always stated that no problem was too small for God's attention, or no situation too big for God to handle.

Whenever she had a problem she couldn't solve, or someone had an illness she could not come up with a cure for, she would pray about it and "leave it in the hands of the Lord".

A specific cure would usually come to her while she was sleeping, or just sitting in her rocking chair by the kitchen window with her hands folded in her lap with her eyes closed, listening to her inner voice.

My Great Grandma was doing what we now call "meditation". If a cure did not come to my Great Grandma and the person's health got worse or they died, my GreatGrandma did not blame herself.

That's Because she was aware that not everyone can be saved, and that she was only working as God's handmaiden. God only worked through her because she was a willing vessel.

When the cure did not come to her, she knew that God was "calling the person home" and there was nothing that she could do to make them well, or keep them on this earth.

As a young child, I watched the positive power of her spirituality and belief system in action. God was by far, the most important relationship in my Great Grandmother's life.

Whenever there was misery or pain in her body, there seemed to always be joy in her heart because of her belief that God was real and alive, and the Holy Spirit lived in and moved through her.

She knew that God worked through her and gave her the desires of her heart. Grandma never forgot to give God glory and praise. In my mind I can still hear her strong, loud voice praising God. I can still hear her giving thanks for empowerment and the ability to heal.

Her prayer went something like this, "God I thank you for the healing herbs which are grown in your garden here on earth. God, you promised that you would supply our every need, and Father you have always kept your word."

"I thank you for sending your son Jesus, who healed the sick and told the world that we could do the same as he had done and even more. Father God, I thank you for allowing me to be the vessel, through which you move and work your mighty healing power."

"Only you could have spoke to my soul and told me which herbs to use, when to use them, how much to use and where to find them. I know Lord God, that I am not worthy of your healing power, but please keep touching my spirit and speaking to my soul."

"Keep my heart clean and pure, and my body strong, so that I can continue to be your faithful servant all of life's long days. God, you know that I only live so that you can use me for your work, and I will always be careful to give you the praise and glory."

"I ask for your continued blessings in the precious name of your wonderful son Jesus Christ, I pray. Amen!" I wonder if I only remember my Great Grandma's prayer because she prayed it so long and loud, that she not only got God's attention, but also everyone else as well.

We all knew when something special had happened. I used to think that perhaps, my Great Grandmother did not leave time for God to listen to anyone else because she was demanding all of his attention.

And mama Birdie was so big and loud, controlling, and passionate in her love for God, that in my eyes God had no other choice but to give her his undivided attention and the desires of her heart.

When she wanted something real bad from God, she voiced her desire, believed that she would receive it and she always did receive it! My Great Grandma Birdie Henderson was a healer.

Her success came from her belief in God, and the basic knowledge that she had of healing herbs. She used only mild herbs, and the plants that are generally treated as food. She understood that food could also be used as medicine.

She was aware that a great deal of love, caring, and practical healing was transmitted from rubbing the body with healing salve, made with herbs, from hot pack treatments with herbal solutions, and through a cup of herbal tea.

Now that you know my family history of traditional healers, it is now time for me to share the healing herbs and practices that I have learned on my journey. This is a mix of healing practices from my family as well as the practices that I have learned in my travels. Enjoy!

Food Used As Medicine

Cabbage was known as "the medicine of the poor" and was used for eczema and varicose veins. Grandmother would grate the cabbage and apply it as poultice to the area.

For those suffering from stomach ulcers, raw cabbage juice was effective in reducing pains and other related symptoms. It was recommended that those in need drink this powerful juice four times in one day and the results would be experienced in a short period of time.

Cabbage was used as a digestive remedy and for painful joints as well as for skin problems of any kind. Cabbage was also helpful for those that were constipated. Results were excellent for reducing fluid retention and for lung discomfort.

An acne lotion using cabbage was also made by using one cup of chopped cabbage juice, strain, add two tablespoons lemon juice and apply to the affected areas until results are seen.

Corn was a useful plant which produces by products like oil fuel and can be processed into flour. Grandma used yellow corn for healing rather than white. The yellow corn is food for the brain and nervous system.

Drinking the water after boiling the corn is very good for measles, because corn acts as a healing agent that cools down the body. Only a few cups of corn water were given at a time. Grandmother thought that anyone could benefit from using corn for food and medicine.

Eating fresh corn right off of the stalk is the best way to get the premier virtues. It is live food. Grandma would dry the corn ear and store it in a dry place for later use. She would roast the corn kernels and grind them for brewed coffee.

She would boil the corn hair, strain and drink the water to tone up the body and organs, especially when swelling of hands and feet were the problem. In all cases the results were outstanding and healing was promoted.

Honey was often added to enhance the taste. Cucumbers were used for beauty rituals and to promote healing and cleansing the entire body and mind. Cucumbers are loaded with hormones.

When menopause begins, hot flashes are experienced. Grandma would give women cucumbers to help. Cucumbers have a calming effect on tension, stomach and bladder ulcers.

She would encourage them to eat cucumbers or make a juice out of them by grating one or two cucumbers together, squeeze, drink all the juice. In Missouri where the sun was very hot in the summer time, so she would cool down the body by drinking cucumber juice.

Cucumber cooler sandwiches were also a favorite. They can be made by peeling one cucumber, sliced thinly, pack on wheat bread and add a small amount of salad dressing.

For relaxation she would encourage men and women to grate two cucumbers, squeeze the juice, and then apply the juice directly to the hair and full body. The old tin tub was filled with water and people were encouraged to relax until the water became cool.

Grandma always used garlic to cook meals and prepare vegetable dishes. The smell of garlic and onions cooking is so wonderful. At least every other day grandma would take chopped up garlic and raw honey. A teaspoon full of this mixture reduces high blood pressure.

Some of my cousins were in their teenage years and developed pimples on their face and backs due to an overproduction of oil and bacteria. For pimples my grandmother would slice aloe Vera leaves to extract the juice.

She would have them wash with warm water and rub the aloe Vera on the affected area. She would have them leave it on overnight to produce the best results. Many of those she encountered had allergies, some of which resulted in hives.

Grandma knew that an allergy was an overreaction to the body's cells to foreign material. Sometimes a breakout of hives would occur from certain foods or it could be an emotional reaction.

As soon as someone saw hives, she would ask them if something was happening in their life, which was upsetting. She would crush aloe Vera leaves to extract the juice and apply to the affected area.

Grandma also encouraged them to drink plenty of fresh water to flush out their system. Sometimes she would have them take castor oil, which would attempt to clean out their system.

When someone came to grandma who was congested and were coughing violently in an attempt to expel the mucus, grandma would give him or her goose grease and flannel cloth to put to their chest.

She would have them go home and go to bed with goose grease and flannel cloth on their chest. She would also suggest that before going to bed, they breathe in some warm salt water.

Another remedy for congestion she would use is to cut an onion and place it on the back of the stove with some brown sugar and take a teaspoon of the mixture from time to time to loosen the mucus.

Since we often went without shoes, we could get athletes foot which is a fungus. This condition would cause the skin to be itchy and flake off between the toes or on the soles of the feet. Grandma would peel one clove of garlic and chop it up.

This was to be rubbed on the itchy area twice a day. Backaches were not uncommon because people worked hard often bending over washtubs or working in the fields all day and would overstrain and pull ligaments, tendons and bones out of balance.

When someone approached grandma that had severe muscular twinges and pain, she would then boil cedar bark in water and have them drink it as a tea three times a day.

In addition, he would give them a light back rub using a homemade liniment made with apple cider vinegar and cayenne pepper. For burns, Grandma would first place the burned area under cold water and then apply aloe Vera.

For severe burns, she suggested that the person contact a doctor. It seemed that one of the children or adults always had a cold. When Grandma saw one of us with a stuffy nose, coughing, or with a sore throat or headache, she would boil fresh ginger root.

Then she would give us ginger as a tea with cinnamon and honey. In addition, she would always use peppermint and horehound candy added to whisky with a little lemon and honey. We would call this a hot toddy.

We liked to have this drink, and we would pretend to be drunk after we would have had two teaspoons full. Babies would get something called colic, which is a sharp pain in the belly of the stomach caused by spasms and gas.

Grandma would crush garlic bulbs, and then put it in warm water. She would also boil cinnamon sticks in water and let them cool, then give to lessen the spasms.

We hated to become constipated because Grandma's favorite remedy was for castor oil and ½ of an orange.

Prunes and prune juice were also used to help constipation. Grandma knew that cramps were involuntary muscle spasms, which could be caused by a number of things such as lack of salt, bad circulation or continuous use of certain muscles.

Sometimes people would have cramps in their neck, stomach, feet or hands. Grandma would make a tea by pouring hot water over cinnamon sticks. She would have the person drink one cup every four hours.

Dizziness is usually associated with an imbalance in the body's balancing mechanisms. When people came with symptoms of nausea, heavy perspiration and spinning feelings in the head, grandma would ask them if they were feeling stress.

Sometimes the dizziness was due to low blood sugar. Grandma would give the person a glass of fresh orange juice and/or peppermint candy. This would help also with an upset stomach.

Earaches were also common and could be very painful. They are usually due to an ear infection and can produce pus. Grandma would put sweet oil on a cotton ball and insert it into the ear.

When we were itching, sometimes from insect bites, grandma would cut a lime and squeeze to extract the juice. She would then wash the affected area with lime juice.

If we had a fever, Grandma would roast dried okra seeds and then wash the seeds. She would boil ½ cup of the mashed seeds in 1 gallon of water for 15 minutes, let it cool, then strain.

We would take 1 cup three times a day after meals. Another remedy was to put vinegar in a basin of cold water and use it as a cold compress on the forehead white with a white cloth. Grandma would make herb oil by taking a handful of any herb and add it to hot olive oil.

When it began to sizzle, she would take it off the fire and let it stand overnight and bottle it in a dark bottle to be used when needed. She made salve by putting 3 ounces of powdered herb into 7 ounces of cocoa butter and 1 ounce of beeswax.

She would blend all 3 of these ingredients together into a covered pot on low heat for 1 to 2 hours. After cooking, she would let it cool. The salve was then firm and ready to use.

Because she did not have a lot of money to spend on herself, Grandma had to use cosmetics which could be easily made from things that we readily found in the kitchen.

Preparation And Usage Of Herbs

<u>Definition</u>: An herb is defined as a plant, especially one valued for its medicinal or healing qualities. Historically, herbaceous plants have been used for flavoring food, for perfumes, and medicinal purposes.

Preparing An Herbal Tea

This is the most common way of preparing herbs. To prepare, steep the herb in boiling water for three to five minutes, so as to give the liquid the taste of the herb. The usual amount suggested is a teaspoon of leaves, blossoms, or flowers to a cup of boiling water.

Strain before using and honey and/or lemon may be added to taste. For general purposes, drink lukewarm or cool, but to induce sweating and break-up a cough or cold, take hot.

DO NOT use aluminum ware in the preparation of herbs. Enamel, Porcelain or Glass pots are suggested.

TYPICAL DOSAGE
1 glass = 8 oz.
1 cup = 4 oz.

<u>Preparation</u>: If told to boil, boil for 5 minutes. Steep for 20 to 30 minutes, then strain. This is for most teas, some may vary. So refer to the specific herb and its boiling time. Just be aware that boiling too long may kill the medicinal properties of an herb.

Preparing A Tincture

Alcohol is used to extract the active ingredients from the herb, because alcohol is a good preservative. Tinctures can be made by combining 4 ounces of cut, or powdered herb in one pint of alcohol such as rum, gin, vodka, or brandy.

Shake daily, allowing the herbs to extract for about two weeks. Allow the herbs to settle. Strain the herbs and pour off the tincture. Extract can also be made using vinegar. Extracts are convenient for external application.

Preparing Herbal Capsules

The herb is dried, powdered, and placed in a gelatin capsule; or mixed with bread to form a pill. Capsules should be taken with a large glass of water to help them dissolve.

This is the most popular way herbs are taken, mainly because it is easy to take and the bitter taste of (some) herbs can be avoided. Capsules can also provide an exact and regulated dosage.

Preparing Herbal Poultices

Medicinal parts of the plant are mashed, or crushed; then heated and applied directly to the skin to relieve inflammation, draw-out toxins, blood poisoning, venomous bites, boils, abscesses, and to cleanse and heal an infected area.

It is recommended that the skin be oiled before applying the hot poultice. The herb can be mixed with water to form a paste. The poultice should be covered with a clean cloth when applied to the affected area. A hot, moist towel can also be used and left on until it cools.

Preparing A Decoction

This is the extraction of mineral salts and bitter principles of plants. Generally, ½ ounce of the herb is simmered in water for five to ten minutes; if it is finely shredded, cook until one third of the water has decreased through evaporation.

If the herb is hard or woody, twenty minutes may be necessary. It usually works best if the plant is soaked in cold water first, and then brought to a boil. Strain while hot.

NOTE: A decoction should generally be used within 24 hours of preparation.

Preparing An Ointment

Ointment (or salve) is put on cuts, wounds, or sores to help the forming of new skin. To prepare ointment, use 3 ounces of powdered herb, 7 ounces of cocoa butter (or any pure vegetable shortening), and 1 ounce of bee's wax.

Blend all three of the ingredients together in a covered pot over low heat, for one to two hours. When it is cool, it should be firm and ready to use.

Preparing A Compress

A compress is also known as a fomentation. This is used when herbs that are too strong to be taken internally may be absorbed in small amounts, slowly, into the system.

This process is generally used for the treatment of pains, swelling, colds, and treatment flu. An herbal compress will achieve a similar effect as an ointment with the advantage of the therapeutic action of heat.

To Prepare: 1 to 2 heaping tablespoons of the herbs are brought to boil in 1 cup of water. A cotton pad, or gauze is dipped into the strained liquid, and the excess liquid is drained off, then the pad is placed on the affected area while still warm.

It is best to cover with a piece of woolen material. When used on small children, the compress could be bandaged in place. When cool, the compress is ready to be changed.

Preparing Herbal Powders

Powders are made from fresh plant parts and mashed until there are only fine particles of the herb. This way, the herb can be taken in capsules, in water, in herb teas, or sprinkled on food.

For external use, the powdered herbs can be mixed with oil, cocoa butter, Vaseline, or a little water or Aloe Vera juice and applied to the skin to treat wounds and inflammations.

Essential Oils And Aromatherapy

I don't know how Grandma knew about what I have come to understand as aromatherapy. It is the ancient art of using concentrated essences or essential oils of certain aromatic plants to promote, enhance or restore physical, mental and emotional health and well being.

She must have had some understanding because she would extract oils using steam distillation from barks, leaves, petals rinds, roots, seeds, stalks or stems of certain aromatic plants, flowers, herbs or trees.

Grandma used aromatherapy for healing purposes especially with the people who were stressed or experiencing the feelings of depression, grief, or feeling anxiety.

Grandma would blend essential oils, such as jasmine, myrrh, sandalwood and rose for beauty, to make the environment or person smell good as well for assisting with spiritual development.

She always stressed to us that there was a tremendous amount of healing power in plants. Following are a few of the ways that Grandma used essential oils.

Aromatherapy And Essential Oils

In my Grandma's day, many African American women could not afford commercial perfume so they would create their own perfumes with essential oils, which offered a natural alternative.

Beside their lovely aroma, natural fragrances can be quite therapeutic both emotionally and physically. Grandma said that synthetic scents were not only expensive but also sometimes offensive and could cause allergies.

As a general guideline, Grandma said that one should add 10 to twenty drops of essential oils to 1/8 ounce of jojoba oil. Grandma felt that jojoba oil was the best carrier oil for fragrances, because it doesn't go rancid and won't spoil your perfume.

She said that you could make your fragrances as intense or subtle as you desire by your choice of essential oils and by the amount of each oil that you use. She stressed to prevent skin irritation you should not apply pure essential oils directly to your skin.

For Women Grandma suggested the following fine flower fragrance. To 1/8 ounce of jojoba oil add 8 drops of rose oil, 8 drops of neroli oil, 4 drops of jasmine oil and 2 drops of geranium oil. These should be combined in a small glass bottle and applied as perfume.

For Men Grandma suggested the following stress reduction scent for men. To 1/8 ounce of jojoba oil add 12 drops of sandalwood oil, 4 drops of clary sage oil, 2 drops of coriander oil and 1 drop of benzoin resin.

She suggested that this be mixed together in a small glass bottle and applied as a fragrance. For quick relief from anxiety, emotional upsets and stress or simply to encourage relaxation Grandma suggested that one inhale an essential oil directly from the bottle.

You could also add 2 or 3 drops of essential oil onto a handkerchief and inhale it that way. She suggested that a relaxing breathing blend be made up as follows:

10 drops of lavender oil, 8 drops of bergamot oil, 4 drops of chamomile oil, 4 drops of clary sage oil and 2 drops of benzoin resin. After blending in a small glass bottle and whiff whenever needed.

Grandma suggested that massage or anointing the body was used as a marvelous way to promote relaxation, minimize muscular aches and pain, subdue stress and tension and treat a variety of conditions in a pleasant and relaxing way.

Besides feeling great, Grandma said that a massage could soothe the nervous system, reduce blood pressure, relax muscles, diminish swelling and help release cellular waste from the muscles, relax your breathing and slow your pulse.

Following are the massage oils that grandma used for relaxation:

2 ounces of carrier oil such as sunflower or almond with 10 drops chamomile oil, 8 drops of marjoram oil. 4 drops of lavender oil and 3 drops of benzoin resin.

For soothing stress she used 2 ounces of carrier oil such as sunflower oil or almond with 8 drops of sandalwood oil, 6 drops lavender oil, 4 drops of chamomile oil, 3 drops bergamot oil, 3 drops of bergamot oil, 3 drops marjoram oil and 2 drops elemi oil.

She would blend these ingredients and then massage them into the skin. Essential oils encourage relaxation and reduce stress. Essential oils are a major part of calming the body and the mind. You can even use oils like peppermint to increase focus.

Essential Oils That Encourage Relaxation & Reduce Stress

BASIL: Basil increases concentration, sharpness of the senses, clarifies thought and calms nervousness. It can either sedate or stimulate. Its sedative qualities ward off anxiety attacks and nervous tension and help relieve insomnia. Its stimulating action fights mental fatigue and strengthens mental function.

BENZOIN: Benzoin has a warming and soothing effect on emotions. It calms and pacifies the mind, eases nervous tension, stress and anxiety and soothes frazzled nerves. Its uplifting effect helps decrease depression and restore confidence.

BERGAMOT: Bergamot oil is refreshing, uplifting oil that acts as a stimulant to balance emotions and moods. It can relieve anxiety, diminish depression and calm anger.

BLACK PEPPER: Black pepper oil increases alertness and improves concentration. It stimulates mental energy, especially blocked energy. It is settling oil that provides a sense of protection.

CEDAR WOOD: Cedar Wood oil eases anxiety, nervous tension and stress related conditions. It also calms emotions and restores energy imbalances. Cedar Wood oil helps maintain emotional composure.

CHAMOMILE: Chamomile oil is calming and relaxing oil and most people prefer its subtle sedative action to harsh, habit forming prescription tranquilizers. It helps create emotional stability and helps combat anxiety, stress, depression, nervousness and insomnia.

CLARY SAGE: Clary sage oil helps restore inner tranquility and minimize the debilitating effects of stress. It calms and relaxes your body and mind. It reduces muscular aches and pains and also restores emotional equilibrium.

REMEDIES

Herbal Teas

Cedar bark tea was used to drink and to bathe in because it is a natural water softener. Cedar bark chips were boiled for tea and/or allowed to simmer on the stove for air freshener, cinnamon and nutmeg was added.

Adding cedar bark tea to the bath water helps with aches and pains. For those with coughs and colds as well as people who smoke, grandma would recommend cedar bark tea four times daily for one month.

In addition, she recommended improving diet using no meat and lots of fresh water to promote healing. When you bark a cedar tree, bark the east and west sides and leave the north and south: the tree will heal faster.

Clean the outer dry bark: chop up the rest and dry in a shaded ventilated area. After all of the moisture is gone, store in an airtight container. Enjoy nature's air freshener when the top is removed.

Brew a strong tea, bathe your dog or cat and rinse as usual. Then using the strong decoction (be sure the temperature is comfortable for your pet) pour all over, don't rinse off.

Herbal Tonic Bath
(For Healing and Special Beauty Treatment)

Grandma was not able to take a bath daily due to the difficulty of transporting water. However, usually on Saturday night the old tin tub was filled and grandma was able to take her herbal tonic bath.

The bath was not only for cleansing the body, but also for relaxing and toning the body. Using warm water, grandma added fresh herbs such as mint, rosemary, pine, ginger, etc.

She would tie the herbs in a cheesecloth bag and soak in the water. She would relax in the tub for 10 to 15 minutes. Afterwards she would rub with a coarse bath towel to warm and stimulate the skin.

African Dry Bath
(For Insomnia)

Using a glove made from coarse material Grandma would massage the entire body before retiring. Grandma said that this would stimulate and refresh the skin.

Bath Tonic
(For Flabby Skin)

As she aged of course, Grandma's skin started to sag. She would steep the following herbs in 2 cups of white vinegar, 2 tablespoons each herb (chopped) of rosemary, lavender and sage. She would then add 1 teaspoon spirit of camphor and ½ teaspoon of powdered alum.

Healing Baths
(For Dry or Itching Skin or Sore Muscles)

To a tin tub of water Grandma would add 9 cups of white vinegar for relief of itching skin or sore muscles. For relief of dry skin, add 1 cup of dry oatmeal to a tin tub of water.

Olive Cream
(For Cleansing)

Grandma would use the following cream for cleansing the skin. Mix together 5 teaspoons of olive oil and 3 teaspoons butter. Keep in a jar in the refrigerator and use as needed.

Liquid Cucumber Cream
(For Cleansing Oily Skin)

Mash cucumbers to extract the juice. Mix ½ cup strained cucumber juice with 1 teaspoon of witch hazel. Bottle it and store it in the refrigerator.

Nourishing Cream
(For Dry Skin)

Grandma washed clothes for a living so often her hands were rough and raw. She used the following mixture to massage into the skin to relieve dryness.

Strawberry Cream: Mix 1-tablespoon lard or shortening and 1 tablespoon of strawberry juice.

Raspberry Cream: 1 tablespoon of lard and 1 tablespoon of raspberry juice.

Lemon Cream: 1 tablespoon of lard and 1 tablespoon of fresh lemon juice.

Orange Cream: 1 tablespoon of lard and 1 tablespoon of fresh orange juice.

Cucumber Cream: 1 tablespoon of lard and 1 teaspoon of cucumber juice.

Magic Beauty Oils
(For Dry Skin)

These were my favorite because they were considered "magic". Grandma would mix the ½ cup corn oil, 1 tablespoon of olive oil and 1 tablespoon almond oil and place it in a bottle.

These oils were used daily and allowed to soak into the skin. She would let it sit for about five minutes and then remove the excess by washing gently and then rinsing with cold water.

Kitchen Wrinkle Cream
(To Soften and Remove Fine Lines)

Grandma did not have wrinkles, but some of the women she washed for did, so she made her wrinkle cream to help them. She would mix 2 tablespoons of fresh cream with 1 tablespoon of honey and stir well.

She would tell the women to apply it to their face and then remove by washing gently. If the skin would feel oily after using creams of any kind, Grandma would mix ½ teaspoon of baking soda to 1 cup of water and then rinse with the skin solution.

Black Night Oil Cream
(For Removing Scars)

There was always a need to remove scars and Grandma would mix 3 tablespoons of aloe Vera juice with ½ teaspoon of vinegar or lemon juice with 3 tablespoons olive oil. Shake well to mix and store in a jar.

She suggested that it be applied nightly for softening and removing new and old scars. Grandma said that it must be used daily for a long time to really work well.

Tender Skin Night Cream
(To Soften and Smooth Skin)

Grandma would melt 3 tablespoons of lanolin (to liquefy) and add 2 tablespoons of almond oil and 2 tablespoons of rain water and beat the mixture until it was creamy. She would store it in a small jar and then use often for the best results.

African Beauty Masks

Grandma would use facial masks to tighten the pores, stimulate circulation and refine the texture of the skin. She said to be sure the skin was clean and then apply the mask and let it dry for 10 minutes or more. Remove the mask by washing with warm water and finish by rinsing it with cold water.

Elegant Egg White Mask
(To Tighten Pores and Skin)

We had plenty of eggs because grandma raised chickens. She would use unbeaten egg whites or beat the egg white of 1 egg until stiff and then spread it over the face. As it dried, it would harden and tighten to stimulate circulation. Remove the water and pat the face dry with a soft towel.

Cornmeal Mask
(For Oily Skin)

Grandma would mix ½ cup of cornmeal with enough water to make a smooth paste. She would apply it to the skin and leave for about 15 minutes to dry. She would remove it with water and pat the face dry with a soft cloth.

Honey And Egg White Mask
(For Sensitive Skin)

Grandma would add a teaspoon of honey to the unbeaten white of an egg and mix. She would add 3 drops of lemon juice and leave it on for 15 minutes. She would remove it with water and pat the face dry with a towel.

Plain Cucumber Mask
(For All Types Of Skin)

Grandma would mix 1 egg yolk with 1 teaspoon of cucumber juice. Apply the mask and leave it on until dry, then remove it with water.

Special Lotion
(Fort Pimples and Oily Skin)

Grandma would dissolve 2 teaspoons of powdered alum in ¾ cup of rose water and then add 1 teaspoon of glycerin and lastly, she would add 1 cup of rubbing alcohol and apply with a cotton pad or cloth.

Honey And Water Hand Lotion
(For Soft Hands)

Grandma would mix and blend well by shaking in a bottle the following:

¾ cup of rose water with ¼ cup of glycerin and ½ teaspoon of vinegar with ½ teaspoon of honey. She suggested that this formula be often used for best results.

Windburn Lotion
(For Irritated and Rough Skin)

It was not unusual for members of the family to have their skin become irritated from the wind. Grandma would mix 1 tablespoon of baking soda with 1 cup of rose water and shake well. She would then apply the lotion with a cotton cloth or pad as needed.

Chapped Hand Remedy

For chapped hands grandma would suggest that vinegar be applied several times a day to restore natural acidity to the skin. She would also suggest that hands be rubbed in vegetable oil or lard.

Nail Care

To harden soft nails, she would suggest soaking them in warm olive oil twice a week and to soften brittle nails she would suggest rubbing them with hydrogen peroxide and then rinsing.

Removing Corns

Many of the people in our community wore shoes that did not fit well and many would develop corns on their feet. Grandma would suggest that they rub castor oil nightly until the corn disappeared or to apply a drop of vinegar or kerosene to the corn nightly.

She also suggested that they might bind a slice of lemon on the corn and leave this on overnight. Or soak a slice of lemon in vinegar and bind the corn overnight.

Birdies Tooth Powder

We often did not have the money to buy commercial toothpaste so grandma would mix equal parts of salt and baking soda for brushing.

Sweet Breath
(For Halitosis)

Grandma would flavor ½ cup of powdered sugar with a few drops of oil of cloves and or the oil of peppermint. Mix well and soften the sugar with a few drops of water to make a paste. Form into small balls and chew to sweeten breath.

Prevention Of Tooth Decay

After brushing the teeth well with salt and baking soda, grandma would give us a solution of weak limewater to be followed with plain cold water to rinse our mouth out.

Reduce Under Eye Bags

Grandma would grate raw "new potatoes" and put them in soft cloth bags. Place under the eye for 15 minutes. Relax while you do this. Repeat daily until improvement is noticed. She would also use grated cucumbers and place pulp in the area once a day until improvement is noted.

Removing Dark Spots
(For Hands & Face)

Grandma suggested that castor oil be rubbed on spots every night until they disappeared. Buttermilk was also applied to the skin several times a day. Equal parts of cucumber juice and lemon juice could also be applied.

Bleaching Cream
(For Dark Spots)

Grandma would recommend 2 teaspoons of zinc oxide mixed with 2 teaspoons of hydrogen peroxide and 2 teaspoons of lemon juice. Mix well. Apply to the skin spots and then leave on overnight. Keep doing this until improvement is noted.

Curly Hair Straightener
(For Coarse or Curly Hair)

Our hair was always a problem. And we kept grandma busy helping us to keep our hard to manage hair beautiful.

Over low heat Grandma would melt and mix well 5 tablespoons of lanolin, 3 tablespoons of cocoa butter, 3 tablespoons of wax and 5 tablespoons of olive oil. She would place the mixture in a jar to harden.

We would apply it to our hair, wait 15 minutes and rinse with a soda solution (2 tablespoons of baking soda to 1 cup of water) and then shampoo our hair.

Anti-Kink Cream
(To Control Curly & Damaged Hair)

After using the curly hair straightener Grandma would have us add the anti-kink cream. This was made up of 4 tablespoons of petroleum jelly or Vaseline and 1 teaspoon of wax with 2 teaspoons of castor oil and 1 teaspoon of lemon oil.

She would melt this over low heat and when it was nearly cool, add a pinch of baking soda and stir well. Store in a jar to be added to the hair as needed.

Peace Bath

Grandma called this her peace bath. To a tub filled with hot water she would add 5 drops of cypress oil, 3 drops of nutmeg oil, 2 drops of lavender oil and 3 drops of sweet oil. She would mix and pour in her peace bath.

Joy Cream

I really don't know why this was named joy cream except that it must have made one feel a sense of joy when used.

She would mix 5 drops of geranium to 3 drops of all spice, 3 drops of orange and 10 drops of lanolin and heat it over a low flame. After it cooled she would store it in a cool place and deep rub where needed to bring one joy.

Hair Wash Oil

This was used to soften hair and soothe the head. Grandma would measure out 2 tablespoons of sesame oil to which she would add 10 drops of ginger to 10 drops of rose oil and 5 drops of lavender oil.

After combining she would rub the oil into the scalp and hair and set it for 5 minutes before washing it out with warm water.

Stress Reduction Bath

Grandma would add 3 drops of lavender oil, 2 drops of geranium oil and 2 drops of orange oil to a tub of warm water and suggest that one soak for 20 minutes to reduce stress.

Stress Soothing Skin Softening Oil

Grandma's formula for soothing and softening skin was to add 10 drops of lavender oil, 8 drops of chamomile oil, 6 drops of sage oil, 6 drops of geranium oil and 3 drops of benzoin resin to 4 ounces of sunflower oil. After combining this oil was to be smoothed over skin after bathing.

Muscle Relief Bath Blend

Grandma would add 4 drops of chamomile oil, 3 drops of bergamot oil and 2 drops of sage oil to a tub of warm water. It is suggested that you soak from 20 to 30 minutes for muscle relief.

Night Time Relaxation Bath

Grandma would add 4 drops of lavender oil, 1 drop of chamomile oil and 2 drops of marjoram oil to a tub of warm water and suggest that one soak for 20 minutes before going to bed.

Soothing Facial Spray

To 8 oz of distilled water Grandma would add 3 drops of lavender oil and 2 drops of chamomile oil. She would suggest that you shake well and spray your face often especially in warm weather.

Skin Softening Splash

To 8 oz of distilled water Grandma would add 5 drops of lavender oil, 2 drops of rosewood oil and 1 drop of neroli oil. After combining she would suggest that you splash on your skin after cleansing.

Revitalizing And Refreshing Facial Oil

To ½ ounce of jojoba oil Grandma would add 4 drops of lavender oil. 3 drops of sandalwood oil and 2 drops of geranium oil. Combine ingredients and apply several drops to clean skin and then follow with the soothing facial splash.

THANK YOU FOR READING

If You Received Useful Tools In This Information, Please Give Me A 4-5 Star Rating!

This serves as a reward for an author. It takes hours and months, sometimes years of no pay to put together books for the purpose of sharing information you see as important to the world.

Please just take out a minute of your time and please leave a quick positive review. Thank you tremendously for taking out the time to read this information and knowledge.

If you really took this information seriously and you applied the key principles into your daily life, I KNOW you are seeing results.

So again, I thank you for your interest in learning and any investment in applied knowledge will always be a winning investment.

For More Books By

Rev. Dr. Geraldine L. Johnson-Carter Visit:

amazon.com/author/geraldinejohnsoncarter

www.ingramcontent.com/pod-product-compliance
Lightning Source LLC
Chambersburg PA
CBHW021545290526
45785CB00004BA/1518